Stoic Healthcare

A Foundation for Resilience in Health and Wellness

Table of Contents

Chapter 1. Introduction

Welcome to an exploration unlike any other - a journey through a special report on Stoic Healthcare: A Foundation for Resilience in Health and Wellness. This is no ordinary health guide; instead, it offers a unique intersection of ancient philosophy and modern wellness. Time-honored Stoic principles are seamlessly integrated into routines and treatments that promote both physical health and emotional resilience. This report is brimming with practical tips, cutting-edge research, and insightful anecdotes. It's a chance to rediscover healthcare, not just as a response to sickness, but as an active, everyday pursuit of resilience and wellbeing. With vibrant language and compelling narratives, this report is a must-read for anyone eager to inspire a spirit of stoic resilience in their journey to holistic wellness. Embrace an extraordinary opportunity to transform your health trajectory and embrace a vitality-filled life. After all, robust health and unwavering resilience could be just a page away!

Chapter 2. Stoic Philosophy: A Brief Overview

Stoicism, as a philosophy, was founded in the third century BC by Zeno of Citium. Since then, its tenets have been adopted by numerous thinkers, across time, providing a lens for understanding the world and humans' place within it. Its teachings resonate particularly for those seeking a strong foundation in life, conducive to resilience and well-being.

2.1. Zeno of Citium and the Birth of Stoicism

After a shipwreck left him stranded in Athens, Zeno found himself in a bookstore, reading the second book of Xenophon's Memorabilia. Impressed by Socrates' character as depicted in the book, Zeno expressed his desire to meet such a man to the bookseller. The bookseller pointed to the Cynic philosopher Crates who was passing by, and Zeno became his student.

However, Zeno eventually broke away from the teachings of the Cynics, forming his own school on the stoa (porch) of the Agora in Athens. It was hence named Stoicism. The Stoics held that all aspects of life were interconnected, part of an overall rational divine plan. They preached the acceptance of life circumstances, the rejection of harmful emotions and desires, and the cultivation of virtue.

2.2. Fundamental Tenets of Stoicism

Stoicism is grounded on a few core beliefs, which include:

Logic as the foundation of understanding: Stoics believed that to assimilate the world accurately, humans must develop good reasoning abilities. For them, logic was necessary to discern truth from falsehood, helping individuals navigate life and make sound decisions.

Physics as the nature of the universe: Stoics perceived the universe to be rational and orderly. They thought that everything in existence was an expression of divine reason, or logos.

Ethics as the path to happiness: According to Stoics, virtue, or moral excellence, is the highest form of goodness and should be the aim of living. They believed that by achieving harmony with nature and accepting the present moment, one could find true happiness.

2.3. The Three Topoi: Practice Areas in Stoicism

Stoics divided their philosophy into three 'topoi' or fields of study: physics, logic, and ethics, each critical to achieving eudaimonia, a Greek term for happiness or fulfillment.

The field of physics discusses the nature of the universe and the role of humans in it. Stoics believed that understanding the physical world and its rational structure is a step towards aligning oneself with nature – a key aim in Stoicism.

The logic aspect of Stoicism involves grounding reasoning in reality. Stoics devised a system of propositional logic that became the foundation of their deductions and argumentations, aiding in the pursuit of wisdom.

Ethics, for Stoics, was the practical application of philosophical principles. They held that the exercise of virtue leads to good character and, subsequently, to a good life. They stressed the significance of four cardinal virtues: wisdom, courage, justice, and temperance.

2.4. Famous Stoic Thinkers

Through the centuries, Stoicism has been embraced by prominent thinkers who have left their unique imprints on the philosophy.

Epictetus, a Greek Stoic philosopher, is best known for his teachings that distinguish between elements of life that are within our control and those that are not. Outlining this in his iconic work, the Enchiridion, Epictetus provides a roadmap for maintaining tranquillity in the face of adversity.

Seneca the Younger, a Stoic philosopher, statesman, and dramatist, contributed profoundly to Stoic philosophy. His letters to Lucilius provide insights on applying Stoic tenets to daily life. Seneca highlighted the value of time, promoting the philosophy as a guide to life, not just an academic pursuit.

Marcus Aurelius, Roman Emperor from 161 to 180 AD, is frequently referred to as the Philosopher Emperor. His Meditations, penned during his military campaigns, provides an intimate peek into his Stoic beliefs and personal reflections.

2.5. Stoicism in Modern Context

In the present day, Stoic philosophy continues to inspire, especially its focus on emotional resilience and acceptance of life's vicissitudes. It's seen not only as a framework for personal flourishing but also as a practical guide during challenging times. Modern behavioural therapies like Cognitive Behavioural Therapy (CBT) have their roots in Stoicism.

2.6. Conclusion

Stoic philosophy acts as a lighthouse during stormy seas, a guide to the harbour of resilience and mental wellbeing. Its links to the healthcare sphere have become increasingly apparent, with its focus on coping mechanisms and holistic wellbeing. We'll delve deeper into this in subsequent chapters, unpacking how Stoicism can be remarkably beneficial for robust health and resilient living.

Chapter 3. The Intersection of Stoicism and Healthcare

Stoicism, a philosophy that emerged in Athens in the third century BC, has proven to be timeless—with much to offer in our taking on the challenges of modern healthcare. Mastering the art of the Stoic philosophy does not merely pave the way to a healthier life. Rather, it ensures the life one leads is of utmost value—physically, mentally, and emotionally.

3.1. The Pillars of Stoicism and Their Relevance in Healthcare

The essence of Stoicism dwells in the core principles—virtue as the highest good, understanding the nature of our control, accepting the dichotomy of control, and living according to nature. Let's delve into how each of these align with the concept of healthcare.

Virtue as the Highest Good: The Stoics saw virtue—or moral character—as the only true good. For them, external things such as wealth, rank, and health are "indifferent". This doesn't suggest they disregarded health, rather they posited it should not be the ultimate purpose. In healthcare, it reminds professionals and patients alike that health, although important, shouldn't define happiness and value of life.

Understanding the Nature of Our Control: Stoicism teaches that our opinions are wholly within our control while external events are not. This resilience-building tenet can be applied in healthcare: our health status can sometimes be beyond our control, but the way we react to it is within our grasp. Attitude and approach, in many ways, complement medical treatments.

Accepting the Dichotomy of Control: This principle is the practical application of understanding control. One learns to redirect time and energy away from things beyond control onto those that can be controlled—which very much applies to the healthcare sector. A disease diagnosis may not be preventable, but steps towards illness management can be undertaken, like diet, exercise, and follow-up visits.

Living According to Nature: For the Stoics, this meant acknowledging the natural course of the world and of human nature—and, therefore, accepting the things we cannot change, including aspects of our health. This could also help healthcare professionals in giving focused care without becoming overwrought with things that are clinically unchangeable.

3.2. Modern Wellness—Stoicism and Self-Care

Within the realm of healthcare, self-care often involves actions we take to preserve or improve our own health, including managing stress, ensuring regular physical activity, and maintaining a balanced diet.

Self-care aligns with Stoicism by recognizing that there is an inherent value in caring for ourselves—physically, mentally, and emotionally. By focusing on what is within our control, we can do much to prevent health problems and manage existing ones. For instance, we can't control the presence of a genetic predisposition towards certain medical conditions, but we can control our lifestyle choices that trigger or worsen those conditions.

3.3. The Stoic Healthcare Practitioner—From Patient Care to Self-Care

Operating within a high-stress environment, healthcare professionals often put their own needs second to their patients. Stoic philosophy acts as a resilience-framework enabling them to perceive and react to stressful situations in balanced, healthier ways. Accepting situations as they present themselves can free clinicians from the burdens of judgment and perfection. This environment of self-care can improve both patient results and practitioners' own wellbeing.

Similarly, the dichotomy of control can help practitioners manage their effort invested in patients. While their ability to treat or cure illnesses may sometimes be limited, healthcare professionals can control their actions, attitudes, and the compassion they bring to their care.

3.4. Stoicism & Patient Approach towards Healthcare

Stoicism can provide a valuable perspective for patients navigating the often disconcerting journey of illness to recovery. Stoic principles can equip them to accept their situation, understand what is in their control, and bolster themselves internally, creating a comprehensive resilience-based healthcare.

Embracing these principles can involve: educating oneself about the disease and treatment options, making lifestyle changes, seeking support, taking prescribed medications, following through with medical appointments, and approaching their situation with acceptance and courage.

3.5. Stoicism to Enhance Therapeutic Processes

Existential therapists frequently use Stoic principles to help patients find meaning in life and obtain freedom from fear, social anxiety, and despair. Cognitive Behavioral Therapy (CBT), a widespread psychotherapeutic treatment, finds its roots in Stoic philosophy.

Using Stoicism alongside traditional healthcare can promote emotional resilience, reduce stress, and support overall wellbeing. Concepts such as mindfulness, acceptance, and cognitive reframing derived from Stoicism can help individuals cope better with physical and mental health issues.

3.6. Conclusion: The Big Picture

As much as Stoicism helps individuals, it can enrich our healthcare system as a whole. By complementing objective treatments with wisdom, resilience, kindness, and acceptance, Stoicism encourages a far-reaching shift—from a 'cure-centric' approach, to one that values overall wellbeing and holistic health.

As we continue to face healthcare challenges, the Stoic philosophy, integrated strategically into our routines and systems, can provide a robust foundation for resilience in health and wellness, ensuring a healthier world for all.

Chapter 4. Principle to Practice: Stoic Concepts in Everyday Health

Many ancient philosophies have transcended time and culture to remain pertinent to our modern lives. Among these, Stoicism stands uniquely suited to guide us towards emotional resilience, helping us cultivate a robust approach to our life, especially our health. Consequently, the focus on the application of stoic concepts to our everyday health will be essential.

4.1. Setting the Foundation: Understanding Stoicism

Stoicism, deeply rooted in the works of philosophers such as Marcus Aurelius, Seneca, and Epictetus, is a philosophy of personal ethics that centers on understanding and accepting the universe's natural flow. It encourages us to cultivate wisdom, courage, and self-discipline, leading us to live a life in harmony with nature, our fellow humans, and our inner selves.

The four cardinal virtues of Stoicism: wisdom(practical wisdom), courage, justice, and temperance(self-discipline) form the bedrock of this philosophy. Each virtue interconnects with the others, creating a comprehensive lens through which we can approach life, and more pertinently, our health.

4.2. Everyday Health: The Stoic Perspective

In the context of health and wellness, Stoicism proposes that health, like any other aspect of life, is somewhat outside our total control. We can eat the healthiest foods, get regular exercise, always sleep adequately, yet, we may still fall ill. Instead of reacting with distress and lamenting our unfortunate fate, Stoicism encourages us to accept this reality. It teaches to focus on what we can control – our attitudes, our responses, and the actions we take towards maintaining our health while treating disease.

4.3. The Stoic Diet: Fueling the Body with Wisdom and Moderation

Consider our diets. Stoicism doesn't prescribe specific foods to eat. Rather, it encourages mindful eating, a conscious decision about not just what we eat, but how and why we eat. Eat to live, rather than live to eat, as Seneca says. The decision to nourish our bodies with wholesome food is within our control. Moderation, one of the Stoic virtues, can be practiced to avoid overeating, to prevent mindless snacking, and to build a balanced diet that aligns with our bodies' needs.

4.4. Stoic Exercise: Harmonizing the Body and Mind

Similarly, our exercise routines can benefit from a Stoic perspective. Exercise should not be a chore, nor should it become an obsession. Rather, it should be a commitment we make to keep our bodies – the vehicles of our existence – in good working order. Epictetus stressed the importance of maintaining the body's condition, not for vanity's sake but because having a fit body could help us perform our societal roles more effectively and discover deeper spiritual truths.

4.5. Integrating the Stoic Philosophy into Mental Wellness

Our emotional resilience is directly tied to our physical health. Stoic principles such as acceptance of reality, focusing on the present, and understanding what is within our control immensely support our mental health. We can choose to view an illness not as a setback, but an obstacle to be faced bravely and wisely, taking suitable actions. This kind of mindset can prevent stress, anxiety, and depressive disorders, or at least make their management easier.

Practicing Stoicism doesn't mean disregarding our emotions. Instead, it equips us to manage our emotional responses better, thereby not letting them overcome our judgment.

4.6. The Role of Stoic Acceptance in Chronic Illness

Accepting the uncontrollable becomes even more crucial when we face chronic illnesses. Stoicism teaches us to realize the transient nature of all things, including life and health. A person with chronic illness could use this perspective to lead a fulfilling life, accepting their condition, working around it instead of continually fighting it, and focusing on their capacity to enjoy life regardless of physical limitations.

4.7. Using Stoicism to Nurture Resilience

Resilience forms the heart of Stoicism. It encourages us to bounce back from our adversities, to perceive obstacles as opportunities for growth, to adapt, and to find contentment in all situations. When it comes to our health, developing resilience means building healthier habits, bouncing back from illnesses quicker, staying positive, and continuously striving towards our wellness goals.

4.8. Conclusion

Stoicism, therefore, is less of a prescription and more of a philosophy of life. It doesn't dictate a set of do's and don'ts for health but encourages a mindful, accepting, resilient, and virtuous approach to caring for our bodies, minds, and spirits. Applying these principles to our everyday health and wellness can lead us to live fuller, healthier, more content, and more resilient lives.

This Stoic approach to health is not just about combating or preventing disease but about leading a balanced, harmonious life – healthily and happily. Let the age-old wisdom guide and strengthen you as you embark on your lifelong journey to health and wellness, laying a strong foundation of resilience in the face of life's unpredictable ebbs and flows.

Chapter 5. Holistic Wellness: Making Sense of Mind and Body

As we embark on this exploration of Stoic healthcare, we must first establish a grounding understanding of holistic wellness. With roots in age-old philosophies and concepts, holistic wellness's central premise recognizes that optimal health goes beyond physical wellbeing – it also necessitates a harmonious balance between the mind and body. Traversing through a narrative of rigorous research, telling tales, and action-oriented advice, this chapter endeavors to dissect holistic wellness's intricacies and showcase its implication for our pursuit of stoic resilience.

5.1. The Fundamentals of Holistic Wellness

Holistic wellness is like a finely tuned orchestra; each instrument, each note, is crucial in bringing forth a harmonious performance. Similarly, all aspects of an individual's well-being, physical, mental, emotional, and spiritual, are interconnected and integral to the individual's overall health.

The physical encompasses everything tangible about us—our bodies and their functional capacities. Eating nutritiously, exercising regularly, accessing preventive medical care, and avoiding harmful habits like smoking and excessive alcohol all contribute to physical well-being.

Taking care of our minds involves nurturing our mental capacities and emotional well-being. This involves managing stress effectively, cultivating positive relationships, and engaging in fulfilling activities.

Spiritual well-being can be found in organized religion for some, or in the purpose and meaning they derive from their lives for others.

Together, these diverse elements form the foundation of holistic health. Wellness, in this context, is not just the absence of illness but is an active pursuit of habits and practices that contribute to overall well-being.

5.2. The Stoic Approach to Wellness

When viewed through a Stoic lens, wellness takes on profound new dimensions. Stoic philosophy, an ancient Greek school of thought, espouses virtues such as wisdom, courage, justice, and temperance, which can guide the attainment of holistic wellness.

The Stoics emphasized that while we might not have control over external events or circumstances, we have control over our responses to them. Applying this to health, Stoics would say that while we might not be able to control the onset of an illness, we can control how we respond – emotionally and behaviorally – to it.

In many ways, Stoic philosophy mirrors current wellness thinking. Experts now recognize the deleterious impacts of chronic stress on health, substantiating the Stoic belief in managing one's emotional response to situations as a key component of wellness.

5.3. The Mind-Body Connection and Its Implications for Health

Modern science has solidified the connection between the mind and body, demonstrating that these two entities are not separate but rather intertwined in intricate ways. Psychological distress can manifest in physical ailment, just as physical health problems can lead to mental distress.

To illustrate, consider the role of stress. When we experience prolonged stress, it's not just our minds that are affected. Stress also initiates physiological responses, such as increased heart rate, elevated blood pressure, and heightened inflammation. Over time, these changes contribute to a variety of health conditions, from heart disease to diabetes.

Meanwhile, physical ailments such as chronic pain or a troublesome diagnosis can spark mental health concerns such as anxiety or depression. The mind-body connection shows that to achieve holistic wellness, we must view our health as a complex interplay between physical and mental wellbeing.

5.4. Incorporating Stoic Principles in Pursuit of Wellness

Given the extensive overlap between Stoic philosophy and holistic wellness, it's unsurprising that many of the tactics Stoics employed in pursuit of a virtuous life align seamlessly with modern health guidance.

1. Respond to what is within your control: Stoics believed in recognizing the difference between what can be controlled and what cannot. If you can't change a situation physically, change the way you respond emotionally and mentally. This principle can be especially helpful in managing chronic conditions and making lifestyle changes.

2. Pursue moderation: Stoics advocated for moderation in all things. This approach has modern parallels in recommendations for a balanced diet, moderate exercise, and avoiding harmful habits.

3. Cultivate inner strength: Stoics believed that individuals could cultivate inner strength to face life's challenges. This aligns well with today's understanding of psychological resilience, a vital factor in navigating health challenges and setbacks.

4. Engage in regular reflective practices: Stoics practiced routine self-reflection to identify areas for improvement and to cultivate gratitude. Modern research suggests that regular mindfulness and gratitude practice can significantly enhance physical and mental wellbeing, thus advocating a key foundation for resilience.

In the next sections, we delve deeper into these practical strategies so you can start actualizing these teachings in your wellness regimen.

5.5. Holistic Wellness: Practical Strategies

If Stoic healthcare philosophy inspires you, you may be ready to incorporate some of these strategies into your own personal wellness regimen. Here are practical ways rooted in Stoic philosophy to advance towards holistic wellness.

1. Practice Mindfulness: Mindfulness, a form of meditation where one focuses on being intensely aware of what they're sensing and feeling in the moment without interpretation or judgment, is a powerful tool in managing stress and cultivating inner peace - the emphasis here, much like Stoicism, is on controlling one's responses instead of exterior circumstances.

2. Cultivate Healthy Habits: Small, consistent changes can lead to big impacts over time. Trade processed foods for whole ones, prioritize physical activity, practice good sleep hygiene, and include activities you love for holistic growth. Here, the principle of moderation applies – you don't have to strive for perfection, just balance.

3. Emotional Resilience: Cultivate emotional resilience by challenging negative thought patterns and fostering positive relationships. This echoes the Stoic principle of managing one's response to circumstances, thereby boosting mental wellbeing.

4. Gratitude Practice: Regularly set aside time to contemplate and list things you're grateful for. This practice aligns with Stoic self-reflection and helps build a perspective that focuses on the positives in life, thereby improving emotional health.

In summary, this exploration of holistic wellness presents a persuasive argument for its criticality in building resilient health. Having traversed through the intricacies of mind-body interdependence and the inherent intersection of Stoic philosophy and wellness, engage with these novel conceptions not just to react better to health adversities, but also proactively nurture your wellbeing to lead a vitality-filled existence.

Indeed, with resilience at the heart of Stoic healthcare, a proclivity for endurance in adversity, and a relentless pursuit of virtues, one can transform their health trajectory. This journey of comprehensive wellbeing, blending ancient wisdom with modern practices, compels us to see wellness not just as a destination but as a continuous voyage. Holistic wellness is not an end in itself but a foundation for cultivating resilience, pivotal to bringing to life the well-orchestrated symphony of mind and body harmony.

Chapter 6. Understanding and Cultivating Resilience in Health

Although applied to differ in form from modern familiarities, the principles of Stoic philosophy converge on one crucial point: the pursuit of tranquility and virtue. From these pursuits, resilience—the ability to withstand, recover from, and grow through adversity—emerges as a foundational characteristic.

Where might one begin to cultivate this formidable trait? Can some of the secrets to resilience be found in our approach toward wellness and in our response to disease? This chapter delves into these questions by examining the intersection of health and resilience, proposing new perspectives and practices based on age-old wisdom and contemporary research.

6.1. Stoicism and Resilience: The Unseen Connection

Imagine for a moment the unavoidable disturbances in life—sickness, aging, or loss. The Stoics argued that it isn't the events themselves that cause distress, but our perceptions and judgments about them. Epictetus, an influential Stoic philosopher, asserted that "People are disturbed not by things, but by the views which they take of them."

This profound understanding offers a compelling framing for health issues. Suppose we can change our views about illness, align our priorities, and refocus on what is in our control. In that case, we craft a more resilient stance towards health and wellness.

6.2. Cultivating a Stoic Mindset in Health

Cultivating a Stoic mindset means focusing on what can be controlled—our judgments, perceptions, and responses. Here's how you can begin:

1. **Embrace adversity**: Adversity is inevitable but what counts is our response to these adversities. Rather than shun challenges, view them as opportunities for growth and learning.

2. **Mind over matter**: While the state of our physical health can influence our mindset, the reverse is also true. Our approach toward, and our interpretation of, our health circumstances can have enormous impacts on our wellness trajectory.

3. **Practice acceptance**: Acceptance is not passive surrender, but active acknowledgment of reality. That might mean accepting an as-is health situation and taking productive steps forward.

4. **Focus on the present**: The Stoics advocated for living in and appreciating the present, rather than anxiously worrying about a future health outcome.

6.3. Resilience in Health Practices

Aside from adopting a Stoic mindset, there are tangible actions we can take to cultivate resilience in our health practices.

Regular Exercise and Stoicism: Exercise challenging our bodies consistently and mindfully, we train ourselves to handle hardship - a staple of physical and emotional resilience. Importantly, through exercise, we learn to work with our limits rather than fight them.

Diet and Conscious Consumption: A Stoic approach to diet might involve mindful eating—being fully present in the act of consumption, acknowledging the source of your nourishment, and practicing moderation. Such consciousness reduces overindulgence and promotes healthier dietary choices.

Rest and Rejuvenation: Stoicism teaches us to appreciate and engage fully with the present moment. This principle can be extended to rest, to sleep without the worries of tomorrow, to recharge entirely and face each new day with resilience.

Stress Management and Stoicism: From a Stoic perspective, stress is a reaction, not an inevitability. It's about embracing an agitated mind's imperfections and focusing on what can be controlled: your response. Stoicism offers an invaluable toolkit for stress mitigation, from mindfulness practices and objective introspection to learning to let go of things outside our control.

6.4. Applying Stoic Practices in Treatment and Recovery

Applying Stoic principles throughout treatment and recovery can fundamentally shift the experience of illness, providing patients with a powerful toolset to confront their health challenges with fortitude and dignity. These may include:

1. **Viewing illness as an opportunity**: Consider your illness as an opportunity for growth and post-traumatic development, fostering resilience.

2. **Separating perception from pain**: Rather than assigning negative connotation to pain, consider it as a neutral sensory experience, minimizing suffering.

3. **Focusing on what can be controlled**: Accept the forces outside your control (like the diagnosis) and focus on your sphere of influence, such as your response and recovery.

6.5. In Summary: The Journey to Resilience

Resilience is not built overnight, and neither is good health. Both require consistent nurturing, commitment, and adjustments along the way. However, with the incorporation of Stoic strategies into daily life and healthcare, we can build greater resilience, achieve better health outcomes, and navigate life's adversities with a sense of calm and purpose.

Just as the Stoics practiced their philosophy daily, making it an enduring part of their routine, so too can we integrate these principles into our health practices. In doing so, we strengthen our ability to withstand, recover from, and grow stronger in the face of health challenges, crafting an active, resilient attitude towards wellness.

As we infuse our healthcare journey with Stoic principles, we could rediscover its true essence: not merely a pursuit to alleviate sickness, but an active endeavor towards resilience, tranquility, and a vitality-filled life.

Chapter 7. Sickness and Stoicism: Ancient Wisdom in Modern Times

Our expedition through Stoic healthcare commences as we tackle the perceivable dichotomies and the labyrinth of interconnected elements between sickness and stoicism. Let's prepare ourselves to break down the barriers of conventional healthcare understandings, and conduct a deep dive into the blue ocean where the wisdom of stoicism awakens a new era in healthcare.

7.1. The Emergence and Quintessence of Stoicism

Long before our current era, in the bustling Athens markets, a philosophy was sown that would flourish into a treasured era of ancient wisdom. Here, a man named Zeno of Citium founded the school of Stoicism in 300 BC. Stoicism is rooted in the belief that our reaction, not the event, shapes our personal experience. It holds a powerful message: Life isn't about what happens to you, but about what you do with what happens.

Here, we unearth the facets of stoicism that play pivotal roles in maintaining health in the face of illness.

1. Self-control allows us to overcome destructive emotions and act rationally.

2. Courage helps us face illness and suffering with resilience.

3. Justice emphasizes the importance of treating everyone, including oneself, with fairness and respect.

4. Wisdom provides judgment and practicality, aiding us in making

beneficial health decisions.

Thus, 'Equanimity in Adversity' forms stoicism's backbone: maintaining composed, fair-minded responses regardless of life's highs or lows.

7.2. Stoicism and the Conception of Health

Stoics conceptualize health differently. For them, being in good health doesn't merely mean the absence of illness but the resilience to confront, adapt, and overcome adversities. It means harnessing our inherent mental faculties to imbibe a sense of tranquility, contentment, serenity, and fortitude, even amid the most testing health conditions.

In essence, the Stoic conception of health accentuates the imperfection of human conditions, accepting and preparing for the inevitable bouts of ill health, and further, extracting virtues out of it.

7.3. Stoic Resilience: A Paradigm Shift in Managing Illness

When we fall ill, despair, anxiety, and turmoil accompany the physical disturbance. But the Stoic approach offers a path to internal peace. It invites us to view illness not as an enemy, but as a part of our human journey – a challenge to overcome, and an opportunity for growth.

A Stoic, staring at the face of sickness, may ask: 'What can I learn from this? How can this situation make me stronger, wiser, better?' It is about finding equanimity when storms hover overhead, learning, growing, and finding tranquility in turmoil.

7.4. Stoicism and the Art of Acceptance

Stoicism teaches us the art of acceptance: distinguishing between what we can control and what we can't. What is up to us is our mind - our beliefs, judgments, desires, and aversions. Everything beyond mind-space, including our bodies, is not entirely up to us. Illness too, in many cases, falls into the latter category.

By this reasoning, while we can't always forestall illness, we can control our response to it. Recognizing the contour of our control cultivates a healthier mental environment and can often influence our physical state for the better.

7.5. Stoicism and Modern Healthcare

As modern healthcare continually advances, the relevance of Stoicism only grows. A growing body of research has found that emotional resilience can dramatically affect the prognosis of chronic illnesses. A study from Harvard University revealed a direct correlation between positive emotional well-being and an increased lifespan in patients facing terminal illnesses.

Moreover, Stoicism guides us to lead a life of moderation, promoting preventative healthcare. Regular exercise, balanced nutrition, healthy sleep – all manifestations of the Stoic emphasis on self-control and moderation, significantly contribute to disease prevention.

7.6. Challenges and Prospects in Integrating Stoicism and Healthcare

Despite the innate kinship between Stoicism and modern healthcare, disparities remain. Many conceive Stoicism as an emotion-numbing philosophy, which is far from its essence. Moreover, the complexity of Stoic principles can be overwhelming for laypersons.

Nonetheless, their integration can do wonders. As healthcare providers familiarize themselves with Stoic principles, they can forge personalized stoic-inspired assistance, while individuals can practice Stoic exercises that build resilience.

Stoicism in healthcare may seem like an unusual alliance, but it imparts invaluable insights into developing a healthy relationship with our bodies and minds. It beckons us towards a wholesome, emotionally resilient life, rich with wisdom, courage, and tranquility, even when staring into the hollow eyes of sickness. This ancient philosophy, thus, breathes fresh vitality into our approach to health and wellness, repaving the path to resilience in an anxiety-ridden modern world.

Chapter 8. Healthy Living: A Stoic Approach to Nutrition and Physical Activity

It was the ancient philosopher Epictetus who said, "No great thing is created suddenly." And this sentiment is perfectly appropriate when discussing a Stoic approach to health. Contrary to popular belief, Stoicism is not about suppressing emotions, but harnessing them to make wise decisions. So how can this practice add value to our understanding of nutrition and physical activity? Let's delve into the principles of Stoic philosophy and their applications in healthy living.

8.1. The Importance of Nutrition in Stoic Philosophy

From a Stoic perspective, optimal health starts with alimentation, focused not solely on the physical outcome, but also fostering emotional resilience and equanimity. Stoics believed that mind and body are not separate entities, but intimately interconnected.

Eating healthfully is not just about looking or feeling good in the present moment, but preparing the body for future challenges. It is an active choice, a selection that promotes life and well-being, demonstrating our understanding that good food is a strategic investment for the future. As Seneca said, "For all things are a scale, and your life hangs in the balance, a life that, while you keep weighing things, slides away."

Here, consider the Stoic emphasis on moderation. Eat to live, not live to eat. Overconsumption and excess are not routes to happiness but to suffering. On the other hand, too much restriction, denying oneself the pleasures of eating, can also lead to suffering.

The Stoic diet is one of balance - plenty of fresh vegetables and fruits, lean proteins, healthy fats, and complex carbohydrates, enjoyed in moderation. It's not just about what you are eating but how much and why.

8.2. Physical Activity As An Exercise in Stoic Resilience

Like nutrition, physical activity plays a vital role in one's overall well-being. The body, just like the mind, needs to be challenged, developed, and maintained through ongoing practice. The ancient Stoics, like the Greeks in general, emphasized the significance of a sound body.

The Stoics saw physical exercise not just as an end in itself but as a means to develop greater mental fortitude and resilience. Exercise is about making the body resilient, yes, but also about developing the willpower and discipline to keep going when things get tough. As Marcus Aurelius said, "The first rule is to keep an untroubled spirit. The second one is to look things as they are and not as they appear."

The best form of exercise is one that you enjoy, can sustain, and that brings you closer to nature. Stoicism often advocates for routines that reflect the rhythms of the natural environment surrounding you. Walking, running, swimming, yoga, even gardening, can be forms of physical activity that embed us in the world around us. Stay flexible, adaptable, and allow yourself to find the joy in movement.

8.3. Stoic Mindful Eating

Stoics practiced mindfulness long before it became a buzzword in modern health and wellness circles. Applying Stoic mindfulness can transform eating from a mere routine or, in some cases, a mindless activity, into a deeply satisfying and health-enhancing experience.

"There is only now. And look at how rich we are in it," said Epictetus. Practicing mindfulness, we savor each bite, fully experiencing the flavors, the textures, and the pleasure that eating can bring. We express gratitude for our meals, appreciating the labor that brought the food to our table.

By slowing down, we also allow our bodies the time to tune in to our real hunger and fullness cues and prevent overeating. We start to understand food as nourishment, appreciate our body's amazing ways of processing it, and foster a more harmonious relationship with eating.

8.4. Active Mindset: Transformation Through Adaptation

The approach to physical activity from a Stoic viewpoint is about more than just the physical motions – it's also about the mind. Stoicism teaches us to adapt, to persist, and not get disheartened if we can't do a particular exercise or reach a certain goal right away.

"Difficulty is what wakes up the genius," said Nassim Nicholas Taleb, influenced by Stoic thoughts. Your body, like your mind, can adapt to new challenges and improve. Write your fitness story one day at a time, one workout at a time, constantly evolving and adapting.

Remember, the ultimate goal of activity is not to achieve a certain physical aesthetic, but to build physical and mental resilience, to be better prepared to meet life's challenges head on, to encourage discipline, focus, and self-control.

By adopting a Stoic approach to nutrition and physical activity, we can not only improve our physical health but also our emotional and psychic wellbeing, leading to more fulfilled and balanced lives. The Stoics understood this intertwining of body and mind and the importance of maintaining both as part of a healthy lifestyle. By integrating these principles into our lives, we tip the scales towards health, wellness, and ultimate resilience.

Chapter 9. Mental Fitness: Stoicism's Role in Stress Management and Emotional Health

Esteemed philosophers of the ancient world held steadfastly that the mind and body share an intimate, pervasive connection. As such, our understanding of healthcare ought to extend beyond the mere physical, encompassing the psychological too. A crucial proponent of this holistic view, Stoicism, holds invaluable advice for those struggling with modern stressors and seeking to foster emotional resilience. Hence, we begin an exploration into the synergy of Stoicism and mental fitness.

9.1. Understanding Stoicism and Mental Health

Stoicism, a philosophy echoing from Athens' academies in the 3rd century B.C., has enduring lessons about managing our mental landscape. Rooting its assertions in the nature of reality, Stoicism proffers that tidings of the outer world are fundamentally neutral – their perceived goodness or badness arise from our interpretations. This philosophy implies radical self-empowerment; we hold the reins of our mental wellbeing, unswayed by external turmoil. Deriving tranquility from this control, we can significantly alleviate stress, anxiety, and emotional distress.

9.2. Stoicism's Four Primary Virtues

Undoubtedly, one cannot delve into Stoic teachings without

traversing its four fundamental virtues – wisdom, courage, justice, and temperance. Cultivating these attributes can consequently foster resilience, balanced emotional health, and a fortified mental state.

+ Wisdom, not merely an academic intelligence, is rather a profound understanding of life's inherent unpredictability and transience. It is the recognition of our limited control, and the power to respond — instead of react — with serenity and acceptance.

+ Courage denotes not just bravery in face of adversity, but also the enduring grit to uphold our virtues, beliefs and inner peace regardless of external pressures.

+ Justice as per Stoicism isn't purely punitive or restorative; it is about striving for fairness and equality in our actions and attitudes towards everyone we encounter.

+ Temperance, the virtue of moderation, urges us against indulgence in any emotion or behaviour, thereby mitigating stress and fostering emotional balance.

Channeling these virtues into our lives will engender a profound shift in our mental outlook, fortifying us against encroaching stressors.

9.3. Living in Accordance with Nature

A critical component of Stoic philosophy is to "live according to nature". In its simplest form, this means accepting the natural order of things—ageing, loss, change—as inherent parts of life, and understanding that distress stems from fighting against this natural order. Meeting life's vicissitudes with equanimity, rather than resistance, paves the way toward emotional health and stress reduction.

9.4. Implementing Stoic Techniques for Stress Management

Practising Stoicism isn't about rigidly adhering to an antiquated philosophy. Rather, it involves applying simple, practical techniques daily to manage stress and improve mental health.

+ **Daily meditation**: Not necessarily a religious or spiritual practice, Stoic meditation revolves around reflection. It could involve evaluating the day's actions, contemplating virtuous responses to stressors, considering your mortality to treasure each moment, or discerning between what's within your control and what isn't.

+ **Negative visualization**: This Stoic technique involves envisaging worst-case scenarios to mitigate the distress stemming from unexpected outcomes. Over time, this method can infuse resilience and erode fear and anxiety associated with unpredictability.

+ **Practising discomfort**: Exposing oneself deliberately to mild discomforts like cold temperatures, fasting, or physical exertion can inculcate resilience and reduce the fear of future hardships.

Embedding these exercises in our lifestyles can yield remarkable improvements in our abilities to manage stress and maintain a balanced emotional state.

9.5. Embracing Stoicism for Emotional Resilience

Emotional resilience is central to mental fitness. Similar to muscle development, resilience can be nurtured and strengthened over time. A Stoic approach to emotional resilience revolves around reframing our perspective of events. By viewing hardships as opportunities for growth and understanding that happiness is within our power, we ensure our emotional stability regardless of unfolding circumstances.

9.6. Stoicism in Modern Psychology

The legacy of Stoicism in modern psychology is significant. For instance, Cognitive Behavioral Therapy (CBT), one of the most widely used psychological treatments, relies heavily on Stoic principles. By identifying, questioning, and adjusting negative or harmful thought patterns—much like the Stoics encouraged—we can drastically reduce mental distress and enhance emotional wellbeing.

Indeed, Stoicism paves a potential path towards improved mental fitness and emotional health. By taking the reins of our inner experiences and interpretations, we can not only manage stress better but also cultivate the resilience to thrive in our unpredictable world. We hope that you, too, find solace and strength in the philosophies of Epictetus, Marcus Aurelius, and other venerable Stoic philosophers, thus embarking on a transformative mental fitness journey.

Chapter 10. Aging Gracefully: Employing Stoicism for a Healthy Lifespan

The Stoic philosophers of ancient Greece and Rome viewed aging not as a disease, but as a natural process. Likewise, in a continuum with these thinkers, we propose to embrace a robust and vibrant vision of aging, utilizing Stoicism's tools to reduce stress, preserve mobility, enhance emotional resilience, and foster an unbroken spirit.

10.1. Stoicism and the Aging Process

In the grand theater of existence, aging is an inevitable act, an integrated part of nature's design, not an ailment to be remedied. According to Stoics, we should not deflect or fear the organic flow of life. To them, aging brings not only physical decline but also maturity, wisdom and, above all, perspective.

Marcus Aurelius, the Roman emperor and dedicated Stoic philosopher, intimated this sentiment, urging one to perceive life from a wider perspective. His meditations unperturbedly reflected on age and mortality, providing guidance on accepting and even leveraging these truths.

Stoicism encourages us to focus on the aspects of our lives that we can control and to accept those we cannot, especially when it comes to aging. The awareness of control and non-control aspects results in life guided by 'amor fati' (a love of one's fate), leading us toward a fulfilled, tranquil experience of old age.

10.2. Embracing Physical Changes

Recognizing and accepting that our bodies change with age is a consequential step in stoic aging. As our bodies go through natural changes, many people lament the loss of younger features and abilities. Stoicism, however, suggests a different approach.

It's crucial to understand that physical change doesn't equate to loss. The changes offer room for adaptation, evolution, and a newfound appreciation of our bodies. To age gracefully, we need to maintain and develop the functions we have, adapting them to serve us in new ways as we age. It might mean transitioning from strenuous exercises to lighter, more regular activities, supporting our mobility and flexibility.

Stoicism promotes the mindset that bodies, just like nature, are in a constant, beautiful state of flux. Thus, accepting physical changes isn't about giving up or surrendering but seeing the opportunity and beauty in the transitioning phase of life.

10.3. Nurturing Emotional Resilience

Stoicism is not about suppressing our feelings but about not becoming subservient to them, about becoming architects rather than victims of our internal world. The transition to older age can stir up complex emotions, and it's natural to feel overwhelmed at times.

Building emotional resilience is one of the most significant elements of healthy aging. The Stoic technique of 'negative visualization' is a powerful way to foster resilience, predicated on the idea of mentally rehearsing worst-case scenarios. This practice equips us to handle adversity better, helping us appreciate what we have rather than what we fear to lose.

Cultivating virtue, the highest good according to Stoicism, is also essential. Stoicism defines four primary virtues: wisdom, courage, justice, and moderation. Aging gives us the chance to reflect and work on these virtues, further building our resilience.

10.4. Enhancing Social Connections

Stoicism highlights the importance of social ties and the sense of belonging which they cultivate. In an age where many older adults experience loneliness and isolation, valuing and nurturing social connections is a way to maintain emotional health during aging. We must see relationships as being mutually enriching, catalysts for wisdom, patience, and shared joys. It encourages us to keep an open mind, be it to new relationships, or to deepening existing ones with acceptance and love.

An array of modern research confirms the health benefits of strong social bonds, including slower cognitive decline, reduced risk for depression, longer lifespan, and improved overall well-being. Stoic practices, such as empathy, active listening, and openness, can enhance these ties.

10.5. Preserving Mental Agility

Contrary to common belief, getting older doesn't invariably equate to cognitive decline. Research shows that certain brain functions, like wisdom and emotional regulation, improve with age. Mental agility can be nurtured in later years as well, reducing the risk of cognitive decline.

Stoics affirm that the mind should be kept active by continual learning. Pursuing new interests, learning new skills, or even engaging in thoughtful discussions can keep the mind sharp. The concept of Stoic mindfulness or 'prosoche', translates into sustained attention and presence in the here and now— which can foster mental agility, improve memory, and facilitate a deeper enjoyment of life.

10.6. Conclusion

Stoic philosophy offers a constructive blueprint to age with grace, converting aging from an anxious journey to a voyage of discovery and appreciation. The acceptance of physical change, the cultivation of emotional resilience, the enhancement of social connections, and the preservation of mental agility are all vital steps on this path.

Let's not forget this wisdom from Seneca: "Old age, especially an honored old age, has so great authority, that this is of more value than all the pleasures of youth." So, as the curtains lift for the act of aging, let us play our parts with virtue, dignity, and resilience, and remain the authors of our life's play, no matter the act or scene. As the Stoic wisdom emphasizes – we can control our responses if not the circumstances, making the process of aging a mindful journey of grace, acceptance, and resilience.

Chapter 11. Checklist for Resilience: Stoic Strategies for Long-Term Health

To fully comprehend and appreciate the intersection of Stoicism and healthcare, it's vital to first grasp the core Stoic philosophy principles. Stoicism, with its emphasis on self-control, mental fortitude, and acceptance, offers a unique way to navigate health challenges. By consciously merging these Stoic tenets with modern healthcare practices, we can foster greater resilience - that ability to bounce back in the face of adversity while maintaining a sense of well-being.

11.1. The Groundwork: Understanding Stoic Philosophy

Stoicism is an ancient philosophy founded in Athens by Zeno of Citium. The school of Stoicism proposes that as we cannot control or rely on external events; we should focus on ourselves, controlling our responses and actions.

The Stoics proposed four cardinal virtues — wisdom (the ability to discern what is within our control and what is not), courage (the ability to confront fear, pain, and uncertainty), justice (treating others fairly), and temperance (exercising self-restraint and moderation). Each virtue is a mental tool in the pursuit of good (eudaimonia), which for Stoics is a life in harmony with nature and reason.

11.2. Stoic Practices for Health: The Checklist

Stoic philosophy can find practical application in our everyday healthcare routines. These practices encompass the entire gamut of the Stoic philosophy:

1. **Understanding Impermanence:** Recognize and accept the impermanent nature of physical health. Health, as with every other aspect of life, is prone to change and decay.

2. **Differentiating Between What's in Our Control and What's Not:** Practice discernment in differentiating between what is in our control and what is not concerning health. factors such as genetics and accidents are beyond our control, but preventive healthcare, regular exercise, and a balanced diet are all within our realm of control.

3. **Embracing Adversity:** Don't resist adversity but embrace it as a core part of life. Struggles can be an opportunity for us to develop strength, resilience and wisdom.

4. **Self-Restraint:** Incorporate moderation (temperance) into all aspects of lifestyle, including diet, exercise, sleep and even in our emotional responses.

11.3. How To Keep up with Your Stoic Health Routine

Maintaining a Stoic attitude towards health and wellbeing requires consistency and regular practice. Here are some methods to make your Stoic practices a part of your daily routine:

- **Daily Reflection:** Journaling or using an app to review your day from a stoic perspective can be a helpful practice.

- **Meditation:** Regular meditation can help maintain mental clarity needed for stoic practices.

- **Physical Wellbeing:** Regular physical exercise as an act of respecting and maintaining our body is a crucial part of Stoic healthcare.

- **Recite Stoic Affirmations:** Regularly read or recite Stoic quotes as affirmations to keep your mindset aligned with Stoic principles.

11.4. Applications of Stoic Principles in Responding to Health Challenges

Stoicism can be transformative in responding to significant health challenges. A stoic response can be achieved through:

- **Adoption of Pragmatic Optimism:** Given the reality of a situation, identify how best one can act within it.

- **Acceptance:** Accept the situation without resentment or self-pity, viewing it as what nature has placed before us.

- **Action:** Take proactive and attainable steps to improve or manage the situation.

Using these aforementioned strategies, you can create an infallible fortress of resilience that will serve you through your life's journey in pursuing long-term health, wellness, and resilience. This is not a one-off approach but an enduring philosophy that can be incorporated into every facet of health and well-being.

By celebrating this extraordinary symbiosis of ancient wisdom and modern healthcare, we create a potent and lasting revision of health – one that embraces resilience as its heart and soul.

* 9 7 9 8 8 5 6 0 9 1 9 8 3 *